This Keto Meal Planner
belongs to:

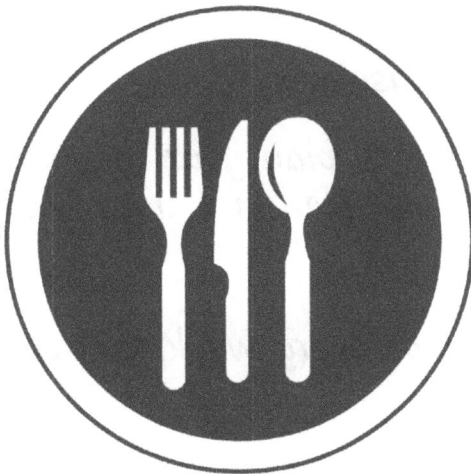

_____

How to use this
Keto Meal Planner?

Thanks for picking up this Keto Meal Planner!

With this food tracker notebook, you will be able to:

- Set your health / weight loss goals
- Plan your daily meals
- Track your progress

Here's how to use it.

Begin by writing down the following:

- Your WHY
- Your GOAL
- Your STATS (weight, waist size, etc)

This is your **baseline**.

Next, it's time to **plan your meals!** This Meal Planner lets you plan and track your meals for 90 days.

At the **start of every week,** you can write down:

- Breakfast ideas
- Lunch ideas
- Dinner ideas
- Snack ideas (yes, healthy snacks are allowed!)

At the start of every week, you will also find space to write down your **shopping list**. This is great if you want to plan ahead!

For **every day**, you can write down:

- How you slept last night
- What you had for breakfast, lunch, dinner and as a snack
- How much water you drank
- Your reflection on the day + what you could improve

And at the end of every week, you'll find a page to **reflect on the week**.

Finally, at the end of every 28 days, it's time to **measure your progress**. Step on that scale and measure the (reduced) size of your waist and hips.

You GOT this!

My WHY

This is why I want to track what I eat and drink:

_____
_____
_____
_____
_____
_____
_____
_____
_____
_____

My GOAL:

Stats at the Start:

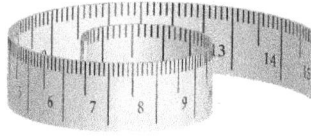

Weight: _____

Chest: _____

Arm: _____

Waist: _____

Hips: _____

Thigh: _____

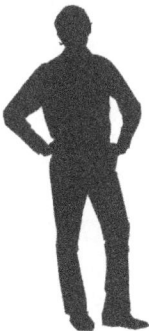
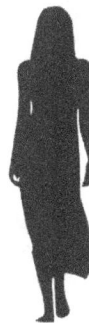

10 Things You Can Do RIGHT NOW

- Make a cup of tea
- Go for a 10-minute walk
- Drink one less cup of coffee today
- Close your eyes. Visualize how good you will feel in 90 days
- Find a recipe for a healthy Keto snack
- Tell a friend about your food tracking plan. Great for accountability!
- Accept where you are in this moment. Give yourself praise for your decision to improve your health.
- Find one thing of amazing beauty. Be still and feel a sense of awe.
- Throw away unhealthy food
- Find your tribe. Go online (Facebook; YouTube) and find likeminded people!

Always
BELIEVE
in
yourself
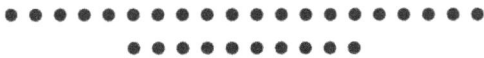

FOOD IDEAS - Week 1

Breakfast:

Lunch:

Dinner:

Snacks:

SHOPPING LIST - Week 1

Day (1)

How did I sleep?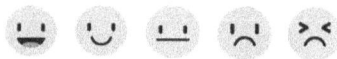

Breakfast:

Lunch:

Dinner:

Snacks:

Water: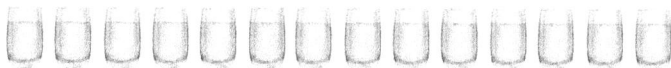

How was my day?

What could I improve tomorrow?

Day (2)

How did I sleep?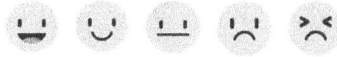

Breakfast:

Lunch:

Dinner:

Snacks:

Water: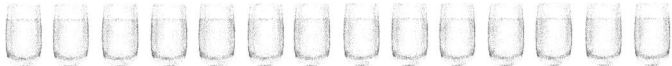

How was my day?

What could I improve tomorrow?

Day ③

How did I sleep?   😀 🙂 😐 🙁 😖

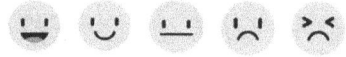

Breakfast: Lunch:

_____   _____
_____   _____
_____   _____
_____   _____

Dinner: Snacks:

_____   _____
_____   _____
_____   _____
_____   _____

Water: 🥛🥛🥛🥛🥛🥛🥛🥛🥛🥛🥛🥛🥛🥛

How was my day?

_____
_____
_____

What could I improve tomorrow?

_____
_____
_____

Day ④

How did I sleep?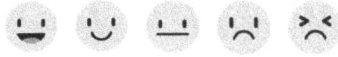

Breakfast:

_____

_____

_____

_____

Lunch:

_____

_____

_____

_____

Dinner:

_____

_____

_____

_____

Snacks:

_____

_____

_____

_____

Water: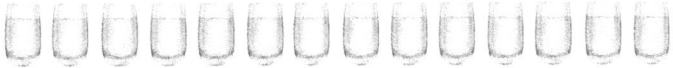

How was my day?

_____

_____

What could I improve tomorrow?

_____

_____

Day ⑤

How did I sleep?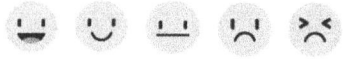

Breakfast:

Lunch:

Dinner:

Snacks:

Water:

How was my day?

What could I improve tomorrow?

Day ⑥

How did I sleep?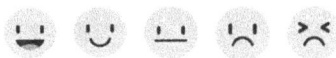

Breakfast: Lunch:

_____   _____
_____   _____
_____   _____
_____   _____

Dinner: Snacks:

_____   _____
_____   _____
_____   _____
_____   _____

Water: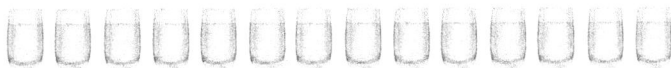

How was my day?

_____
_____
_____

What could I improve tomorrow?

_____
_____
_____

Day ⑦

How did I sleep?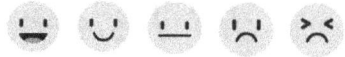

Breakfast:

_____
_____
_____
_____

Lunch:

_____
_____
_____
_____

Dinner:

_____
_____
_____

Snacks:

_____
_____
_____

Water: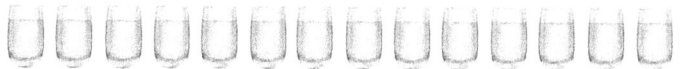

How was my day?

_____
_____

What could I improve tomorrow?

_____
_____
_____

Reflection - Week 1

How was my week?

_____

_____

_____

_____

What lesson did I learn?

_____

_____

_____

_____

What change would make next
week (even) better?

_____

_____

_____

_____

FOOD IDEAS - Week 2

Breakfast:

Lunch:

Dinner:

Snacks:

SHOPPING LIST - Week 2

THE
BEST WAY
to
PREDICT
the
◄future►
is
TO create IT

Day 8

How did I sleep?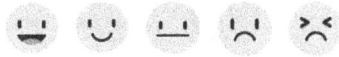

Breakfast:

_____

_____

_____

_____

Lunch:

_____

_____

_____

_____

Dinner:

_____

_____

_____

Snacks:

_____

_____

_____

Water: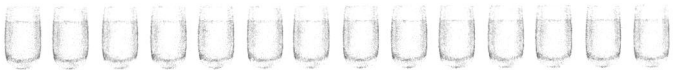

How was my day?

_____

_____

What could I improve tomorrow?

_____

_____

Day ⑨

How did I sleep?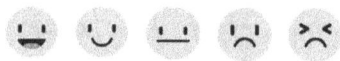

Breakfast:

Lunch:

Dinner:

Snacks:

Water: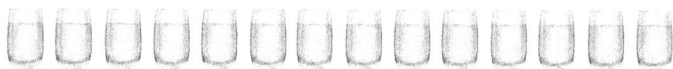

How was my day?

What could I improve tomorrow?

How did I sleep?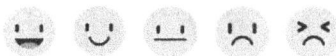

Breakfast:

_____
_____
_____
_____

Lunch:

_____
_____
_____
_____

Dinner:

_____
_____
_____
_____

Snacks:

_____
_____
_____
_____

Water: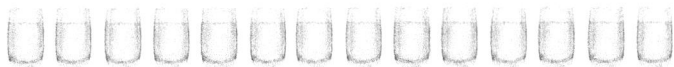

How was my day?

_____
_____
_____

What could I improve tomorrow?

_____
_____
_____

Day (11)

How did I sleep?　😛 🙂 😐 😟 😣

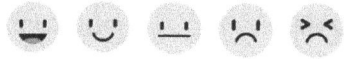

Breakfast:　　　　　　　Lunch:

_____　_____
_____　_____
_____　_____
_____　_____

Dinner:　　　　　　　　Snacks:

_____　_____
_____　_____
_____　_____
_____　_____

Water: 　⊔⊔⊔⊔⊔⊔⊔⊔⊔⊔⊔⊔⊔⊔⊔⊔

How was my day?

_____
_____
_____

What could I improve tomorrow?

_____
_____
_____

Day ⑫

How did I sleep?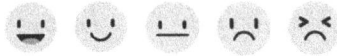

Breakfast: Lunch:

_____   _____
_____   _____
_____   _____
_____   _____

Dinner: Snacks:

_____   _____
_____   _____
_____   _____
_____   _____

Water: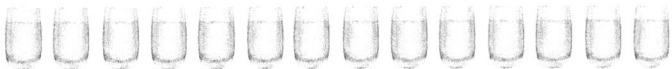

How was my day?

_____
_____
_____

What could I improve tomorrow?

_____
_____
_____

Day 13

How did I sleep? 🙂 🙂 😐 🙁 😣

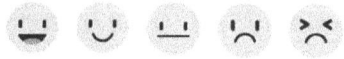

Breakfast:

_____

_____

_____

_____

_____

Lunch:

_____

_____

_____

_____

Dinner:

_____

_____

_____

_____

Snacks:

_____

_____

_____

_____

Water: ⎍⎍⎍⎍⎍⎍⎍⎍⎍⎍⎍⎍⎍⎍

How was my day?

_____

_____

_____

What could I improve tomorrow?

_____

_____

_____

Day (14)

How did I sleep?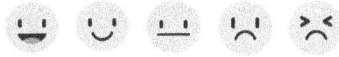

Breakfast:

_____
_____
_____
_____

Lunch:

_____
_____
_____
_____

Dinner:

_____
_____
_____
_____

Snacks:

_____
_____
_____
_____

Water: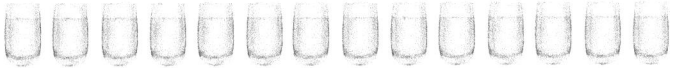

How was my day?

_____
_____
_____

What could I improve tomorrow?

_____
_____

Reflection - Week 2

How was my week?

_____

_____

_____

_____

_____

What lesson did I learn?

_____

_____

_____

_____

What change would make next
week (even) better?

_____

_____

_____

_____

★

DON'T SAY

≈≈≈ I ≈≈≈

WISH

Say

I WILL

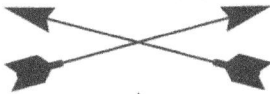

★

FOOD IDEAS - Week 3

Breakfast:

Lunch:

Dinner:

Snacks:

SHOPPING LIST - Week 3

Day (15)

How did I sleep?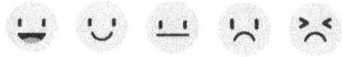

Breakfast: Lunch:

_____   _____
_____   _____
_____   _____
_____   _____

Dinner: Snacks:

_____   _____
_____   _____
_____   _____

Water: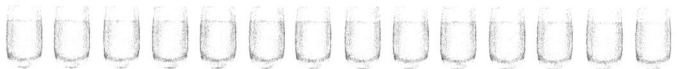

How was my day?

_____
_____
_____

What could I improve tomorrow?

_____
_____
_____

Day (16)

How did I sleep?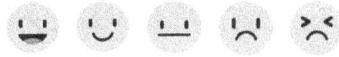

Breakfast:

Lunch:

_____

_____

_____

_____

Dinner:

Snacks:

_____

_____

_____

Water: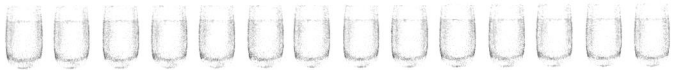

How was my day?

_____

_____

What could I improve tomorrow?

_____

_____

Day (17)

How did I sleep?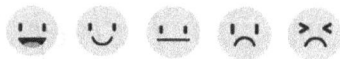

Breakfast:

_____
_____
_____
_____

Lunch:

_____
_____
_____
_____

Dinner:

_____
_____
_____

Snacks:

_____
_____
_____

Water: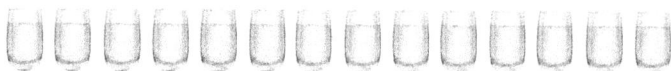

How was my day?

_____
_____
_____

What could I improve tomorrow?

_____
_____
_____

Day ⑱

How did I sleep?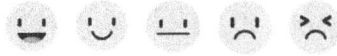

Breakfast:

_____

_____

_____

_____

Lunch:

_____

_____

_____

Dinner:

_____

_____

_____

Snacks:

_____

_____

_____

Water: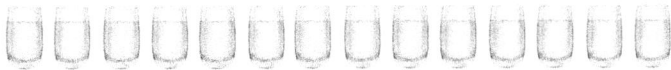

How was my day?

_____

_____

_____

What could I improve tomorrow?

_____

_____

_____

Day (19)

How did I sleep? 🙂 🙂 😐 🙁 😖

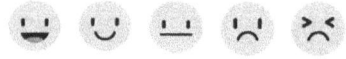

Breakfast:

_____
_____
_____
_____

Lunch:

_____
_____
_____
_____

Dinner:

_____
_____
_____
_____

Snacks:

_____
_____
_____
_____

Water: ⊔⊔⊔⊔⊔⊔⊔⊔⊔⊔⊔⊔⊔⊔⊔⊔

How was my day?

_____
_____
_____

What could I improve tomorrow?

_____
_____
_____

Day (20)

How did I sleep?   😀 🙂 😐 🙁 😣

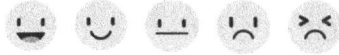

Breakfast:

_____
_____
_____
_____

Lunch:

_____
_____
_____
_____

Dinner:

_____
_____
_____
_____

Snacks:

_____
_____
_____
_____

Water: ⊔⊔⊔⊔⊔⊔⊔⊔⊔⊔⊔⊔⊔⊔⊔

How was my day?

_____
_____
_____

What could I improve tomorrow?

_____
_____
_____

Day ㉑

How did I sleep?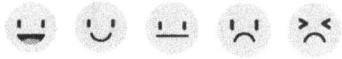

Breakfast:

_____

_____

_____

_____

Lunch:

_____

_____

_____

_____

Dinner:

_____

_____

_____

_____

Snacks:

_____

_____

_____

_____

Water: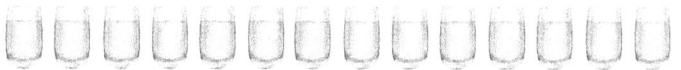

How was my day?

_____

_____

_____

What could I improve tomorrow?

_____

_____

_____

Reflection - Week 3

How was my week?

_____

_____

_____

_____

_____

What lesson did I learn?

_____

_____

_____

_____

_____

What change would make next week (even) better?

_____

_____

_____

_____

_____

FOOD IDEAS - Week 4

Breakfast:

Lunch:

Dinner:

Snacks:

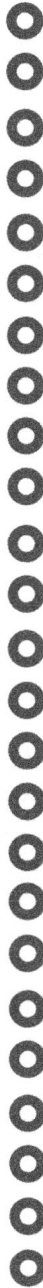

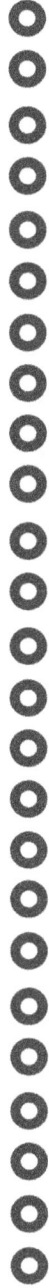

SHOPPING LIST - Week 4

Day (22)

How did I sleep?

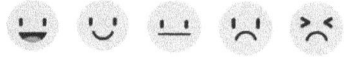

Breakfast:

Lunch:

Dinner:

Snacks:

Water:

How was my day?

What could I improve tomorrow?

Day (23)

How did I sleep?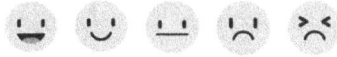

Breakfast:

Lunch:

Dinner:

Snacks:

Water: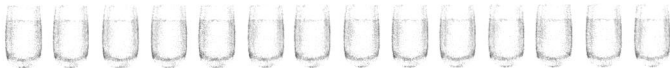

How was my day?

What could I improve tomorrow?

Day (24)

How did I sleep?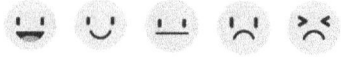

Breakfast:

_____
_____
_____
_____

Lunch:

_____
_____
_____
_____

Dinner:

_____
_____
_____

Snacks:

_____
_____
_____

Water: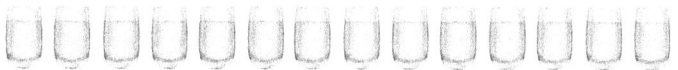

How was my day?

_____
_____
_____

What could I improve tomorrow?

_____
_____
_____

Day (25)

How did I sleep?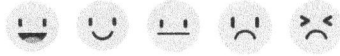

Breakfast: Lunch:

_____   _____
_____   _____
_____   _____
_____   _____

Dinner: Snacks:

_____   _____
_____   _____
_____   _____
_____   _____

Water: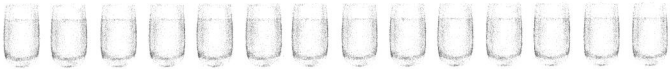

How was my day?

_____
_____

What could I improve tomorrow?

_____
_____

Day (26)

How did I sleep?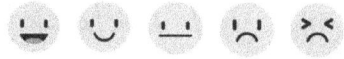

Breakfast:

_____
_____
_____
_____

Lunch:

_____
_____
_____
_____

Dinner:

_____
_____
_____
_____

Snacks:

_____
_____
_____
_____

Water: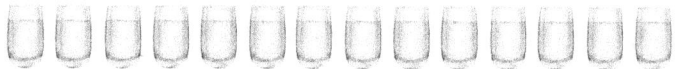

How was my day?

_____
_____
_____

What could I improve tomorrow?

_____
_____
_____

How did I sleep?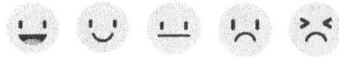

Breakfast:

Lunch:

Dinner:

Snacks:

Water: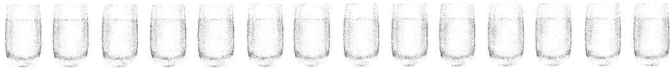

How was my day?

What could I improve tomorrow?

Day 28

How did I sleep? 😀 🙂 😐 🙁 😣

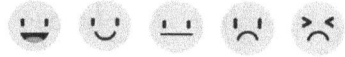

Breakfast:

_____
_____
_____
_____

Lunch:

_____
_____
_____
_____

Dinner:

_____
_____
_____
_____

Snacks:

_____
_____
_____

Water: ⊔⊔⊔⊔⊔⊔⊔⊔⊔⊔⊔⊔⊔⊔⊔

How was my day?

_____
_____
_____

What could I improve tomorrow?

_____
_____
_____

Reflection - Week 4

How was my week?

_____

_____

_____

_____

_____

What lesson did I learn?

_____

_____

_____

_____

What change would make next week (even) better?

_____

_____

_____

_____

Stats After 4 Weeks:

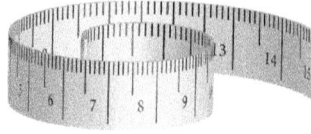

Weight: _____

Chest: _____

Arm: _____

Waist: _____

Hips: _____

Thigh: _____

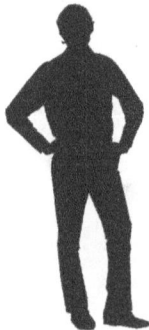

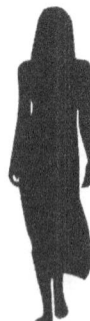

Opportunity

doesn't knock,

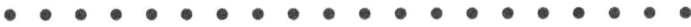

build

@

DOOR

FOOD IDEAS - Week 5

Breakfast:

Lunch:

Dinner:

Snacks:

SHOPPING LIST - Week 5

Day (29)

How did I sleep?　😀 🙂 😐 🙁 😣

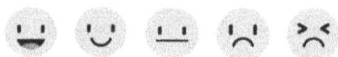

Breakfast:　　　　　Lunch:

_____　_____
_____　_____
_____　_____
_____　_____

Dinner:　　　　　　Snacks:

_____　_____
_____　_____
_____　_____
_____　_____

Water: ⏧⏧⏧⏧⏧⏧⏧⏧⏧⏧⏧⏧⏧

How was my day?

_____
_____
_____

What could I improve tomorrow?

_____
_____
_____

How did I sleep? 😀 🙂 😐 🙁 😣

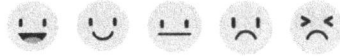

Breakfast:

_____
_____
_____
_____

Lunch:

_____
_____
_____
_____

Dinner:

_____
_____
_____

Snacks:

_____
_____
_____

Water: 🥛🥛🥛🥛🥛🥛🥛🥛🥛🥛🥛🥛🥛🥛

How was my day?

_____
_____
_____

What could I improve tomorrow?

_____
_____

Day (31)

How did I sleep?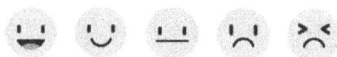

Breakfast: Lunch:

_____   _____
_____   _____
_____   _____
_____   _____

Dinner: Snacks:

_____   _____
_____   _____
_____   _____

Water: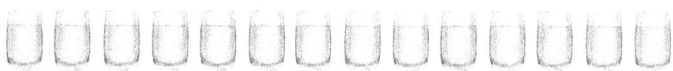

How was my day?

_____
_____
_____

What could I improve tomorrow?

_____
_____
_____

Day (32)

How did I sleep?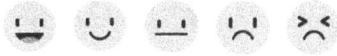

Breakfast:

Lunch:

_____
_____
_____
_____

_____
_____
_____
_____

Dinner:

Snacks:

_____
_____
_____
_____

_____
_____
_____
_____

Water: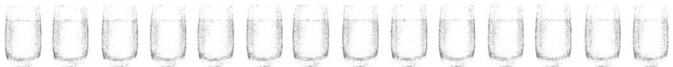

How was my day?

_____
_____
_____

What could I improve tomorrow?

_____
_____
_____

Day ㉝

How did I sleep?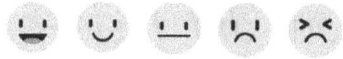

Breakfast:

_____
_____
_____
_____

Lunch:

_____
_____
_____
_____

Dinner:

_____
_____
_____

Snacks:

_____
_____
_____
_____

Water: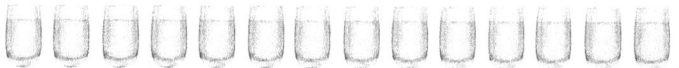

How was my day?

_____
_____
_____

What could I improve tomorrow?

_____
_____
_____

How did I sleep? 😀 🙂 😐 🙁 😣

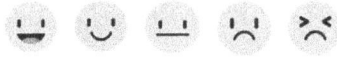

Breakfast: Lunch:

_____   _____
_____   _____
_____   _____
_____   _____

Dinner: Snacks:

_____   _____
_____   _____
_____   _____
_____   _____

Water: ⊔⊔⊔⊔⊔⊔⊔⊔⊔⊔⊔⊔⊔⊔

How was my day?

_____
_____
_____

What could I improve tomorrow?

_____
_____
_____

Day (35)

How did I sleep?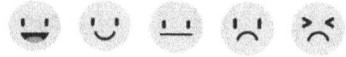

Breakfast:

_____
_____
_____
_____

Lunch:

_____
_____
_____
_____

Dinner:

_____
_____
_____
_____

Snacks:

_____
_____
_____
_____

Water: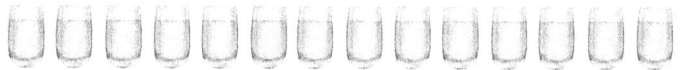

How was my day?

_____
_____
_____

What could I improve tomorrow?

_____
_____
_____

Reflection - Week 5

How was my week?

_____

_____

_____

_____

What lesson did I learn?

_____

_____

_____

_____

What change would make next week (even) better?

_____

_____

_____

_____

FOOD IDEAS - Week 6

Breakfast:

Lunch:

Dinner:

Snacks:

SHOPPING LIST - Week 6

Day (36)

How did I sleep?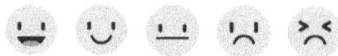

Breakfast:

_____
_____
_____
_____

Lunch:

_____
_____
_____
_____

Dinner:

_____
_____
_____

Snacks:

_____
_____
_____

Water: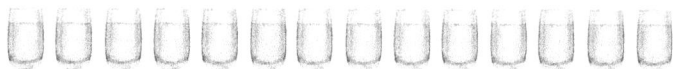

How was my day?

_____
_____
_____

What could I improve tomorrow?

_____
_____
_____

Day (37)

How did I sleep?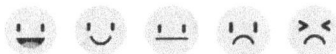

Breakfast: Lunch:

_____   _____
_____   _____
_____   _____
_____   _____

Dinner: Snacks:

_____   _____
_____   _____
_____   _____

Water: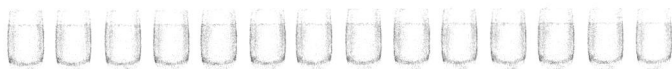

How was my day?

_____
_____
_____

What could I improve tomorrow?

_____
_____
_____

Day (38)

How did I sleep?

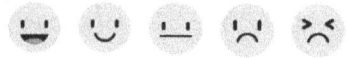

Breakfast:

Lunch:

Dinner:

Snacks:

Water:

How was my day?

What could I improve tomorrow?

How did I sleep?   😀 🙂 😐 🙁 😣

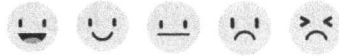

Breakfast: Lunch:

_____   _____
_____   _____
_____   _____
_____   _____
_____   _____

Dinner: Snacks:

_____   _____
_____   _____
_____   _____
_____   _____

Water: ⎕⎕⎕⎕⎕⎕⎕⎕⎕⎕⎕⎕⎕⎕

How was my day?

_____
_____
_____

What could I improve tomorrow?

_____
_____

Day (40)

How did I sleep?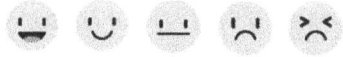

Breakfast:

_____
_____
_____
_____

Lunch:

_____
_____
_____
_____

Dinner:

_____
_____
_____
_____

Snacks:

_____
_____
_____
_____

Water: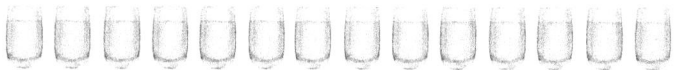

How was my day?

_____
_____
_____

What could I improve tomorrow?

_____
_____
_____

Day (41)

How did I sleep?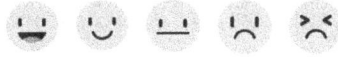

Breakfast:

Lunch:

Dinner:

Snacks:

Water: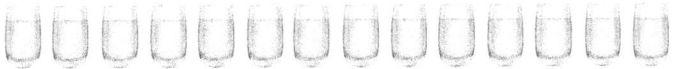

How was my day?

What could I improve tomorrow?

Day (42)

How did I sleep?   😀 🙂 😐 🙁 😣

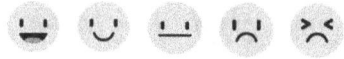

Breakfast:

_____
_____
_____
_____

Lunch:

_____
_____
_____
_____

Dinner:

_____
_____
_____

Snacks:

_____
_____
_____

Water: 🥤🥤🥤🥤🥤🥤🥤🥤🥤🥤🥤🥤🥤🥤

How was my day?

_____
_____
_____

What could I improve tomorrow?

_____
_____
_____

Reflection - Week 6

How was my week?

_____

_____

_____

_____

What lesson did I learn?

_____

_____

_____

What change would make next
week (even) better?

_____

_____

_____

_____

FOOD IDEAS - Week 7

Breakfast:

Lunch:

Dinner:

Snacks:

SHOPPING LIST - Week 7

Day (43)

How did I sleep?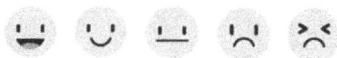

Breakfast:

Lunch:

Dinner:

Snacks:

Water: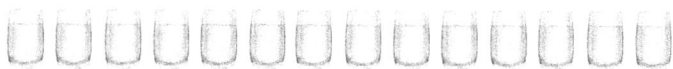

How was my day?

What could I improve tomorrow?

Day (44)

How did I sleep?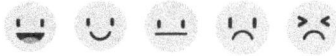

Breakfast:

_____
_____
_____
_____

Lunch:

_____
_____
_____
_____

Dinner:

_____
_____
_____

Snacks:

_____
_____
_____

Water: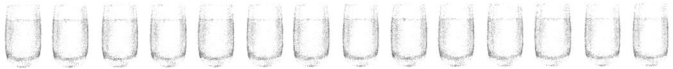

How was my day?

_____
_____
_____

What could I improve tomorrow?

_____
_____

Day 45

How did I sleep? 😛 🙂 😐 😠 😣

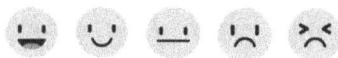

Breakfast:

_____
_____
_____
_____

Lunch:

_____
_____
_____
_____

Dinner:

_____
_____
_____

Snacks:

_____
_____
_____

Water: 🥛🥛🥛🥛🥛🥛🥛🥛🥛🥛🥛🥛

How was my day?

_____
_____
_____

What could I improve tomorrow?

_____
_____
_____

Day (46)

How did I sleep?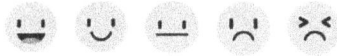

Breakfast:

_____
_____
_____
_____

Lunch:

_____
_____
_____
_____

Dinner:

_____
_____
_____
_____

Snacks:

_____
_____
_____
_____

Water: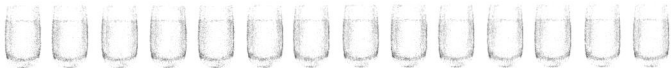

How was my day?

_____
_____
_____

What could I improve tomorrow?

_____
_____
_____

Day 47

How did I sleep?

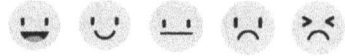

Breakfast:

Lunch:

Dinner:

Snacks:

Water:

How was my day?

What could I improve tomorrow?

How did I sleep?   🙂 🙂 😐 🙁 😣

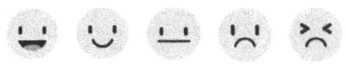

Breakfast: Lunch:

_____   _____
_____   _____
_____   _____
_____   _____

Dinner: Snacks:

_____   _____
_____   _____
_____   _____

Water: ⎕⎕⎕⎕⎕⎕⎕⎕⎕⎕⎕⎕⎕⎕

How was my day?

_____
_____
_____

What could I improve tomorrow?

_____
_____
_____

Day (49)

How did I sleep?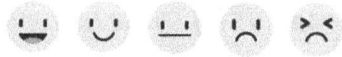

Breakfast:

Lunch:

Dinner:

Snacks:

Water: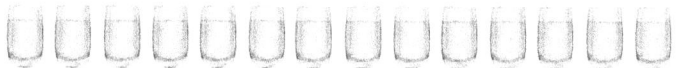

How was my day?

What could I improve tomorrow?

Reflection - Week 7

How was my week?

_____

_____

_____

_____

_____

What lesson did I learn?

_____

_____

_____

_____

_____

What change would make next week (even) better?

_____

_____

_____

_____

FOOD IDEAS - Week 8

Breakfast:

Lunch:

Dinner:

Snacks:

SHOPPING LIST - Week 8

Day (50)

How did I sleep?   😀 🙂 😐 🙁 😣

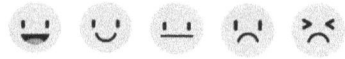

Breakfast:
_____
_____
_____
_____

Lunch:
_____
_____
_____
_____

Dinner:
_____
_____
_____
_____

Snacks:
_____
_____
_____
_____

Water: 🥛🥛🥛🥛🥛🥛🥛🥛🥛🥛🥛🥛🥛🥛

How was my day?
_____
_____
_____

What could I improve tomorrow?
_____
_____
_____

How did I sleep?

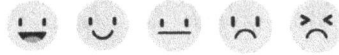

Breakfast:

_____
_____
_____
_____

Lunch:

_____
_____
_____
_____

Dinner:

_____
_____
_____
_____

Snacks:

_____
_____
_____
_____

Water:

How was my day?

_____
_____
_____

What could I improve tomorrow?

_____
_____
_____

Day 52

How did I sleep?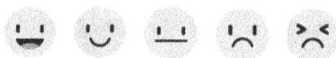

Breakfast:

Lunch:

Dinner:

Snacks:

Water: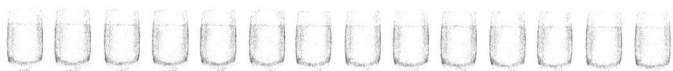

How was my day?

What could I improve tomorrow?

Day (53)

How did I sleep?   😀 🙂 😐 🙁 😣

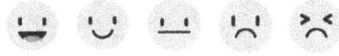

Breakfast:

_____
_____
_____
_____

Lunch:

_____
_____
_____
_____

Dinner:

_____
_____
_____
_____

Snacks:

_____
_____
_____
_____

Water: 🥛🥛🥛🥛🥛🥛🥛🥛🥛🥛🥛🥛🥛🥛🥛

How was my day?

_____
_____
_____

What could I improve tomorrow?

_____
_____
_____

Day (54)

How did I sleep?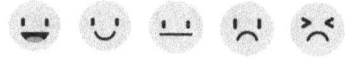

Breakfast:

_____
_____
_____
_____

Lunch:

_____
_____
_____
_____

Dinner:

_____
_____
_____
_____

Snacks:

_____
_____
_____
_____

Water: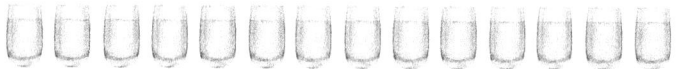

How was my day?

_____
_____
_____

What could I improve tomorrow?

_____
_____
_____

Day 55

How did I sleep? 😋 🙂 😐 🙁 😣

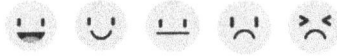

Breakfast:

_____
_____
_____
_____

Lunch:

_____
_____
_____

Dinner:

_____
_____
_____

Snacks:

_____
_____
_____

Water: ⊔⊔⊔⊔⊔⊔⊔⊔⊔⊔⊔⊔⊔⊔

How was my day?

_____
_____
_____

What could I improve tomorrow?

_____
_____
_____

Day 56

How did I sleep? 😀 🙂 😐 🙁 😣

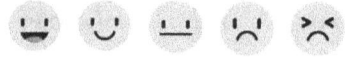

Breakfast:

_____

_____

_____

_____

Lunch:

_____

_____

_____

_____

Dinner:

_____

_____

_____

_____

Snacks:

_____

_____

_____

_____

Water: 🥛🥛🥛🥛🥛🥛🥛🥛🥛🥛🥛🥛🥛🥛🥛

How was my day?

_____

_____

_____

What could I improve tomorrow?

_____

_____

_____

Reflection - Week 8

How was my week?

What lesson did I learn?

What change would make next
week (even) better?

Stats After 8 Weeks:

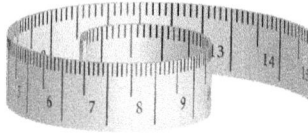

Weight: _____

Chest: _____

Arm: _____

Waist: _____

Hips: _____

Thigh: _____

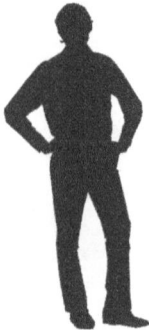

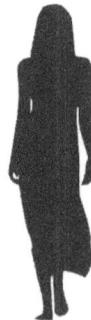

SUCCESS

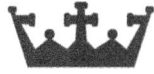 is a

STATE

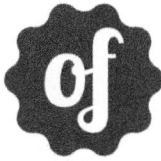

MIND

FOOD IDEAS - Week 9

Breakfast:

Lunch:

Dinner:

Snacks:

SHOPPING LIST - Week 9

Day (57)

How did I sleep?   😀 🙂 😐 🙁 😣

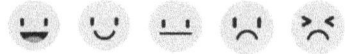

Breakfast:

_____

_____

_____

_____

Lunch:

_____

_____

_____

_____

Dinner:

_____

_____

_____

_____

Snacks:

_____

_____

_____

_____

Water: ⊔⊔⊔⊔⊔⊔⊔⊔⊔⊔⊔⊔

How was my day?

_____

_____

_____

What could I improve tomorrow?

_____

_____

_____

How did I sleep? 😛 🙂 😐 🙁 😣

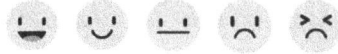

Breakfast:

_____
_____
_____
_____

Lunch:

_____
_____
_____
_____

Dinner:

_____
_____
_____

Snacks:

_____
_____
_____

Water: ⊔⊔⊔⊔⊔⊔⊔⊔⊔⊔⊔⊔⊔⊔

How was my day?

_____
_____
_____

What could I improve tomorrow?

_____
_____
_____

Day 59

How did I sleep?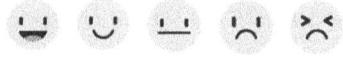

Breakfast:

_____

_____

_____

_____

Lunch:

_____

_____

_____

_____

Dinner:

_____

_____

_____

_____

Snacks:

_____

_____

_____

_____

Water: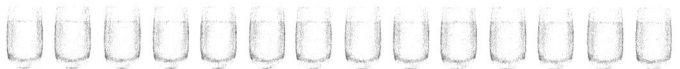

How was my day?

_____

_____

_____

What could I improve tomorrow?

_____

_____

_____

How did I sleep? 😀 🙂 😐 😟 😣

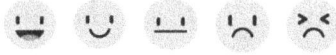

Breakfast:

Lunch:

Dinner:

Snacks:

Water:

How was my day?

What could I improve tomorrow?

Day (61)

How did I sleep?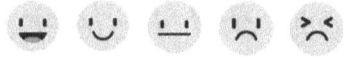

Breakfast:

_____
_____
_____
_____

Lunch:

_____
_____
_____
_____

Dinner:

_____
_____
_____
_____

Snacks:

_____
_____
_____
_____

Water: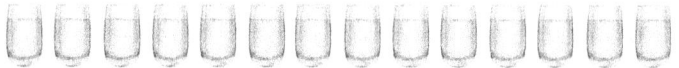

How was my day?

_____
_____
_____

What could I improve tomorrow?

_____
_____
_____

How did I sleep?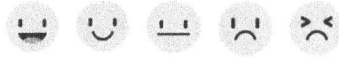

Breakfast:

Lunch:

Dinner:

Snacks:

Water: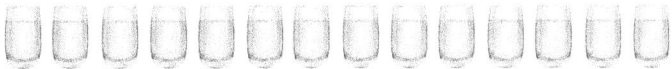

How was my day?

What could I improve tomorrow?

Day 63

How did I sleep? 😃 🙂 😐 🙁 😣

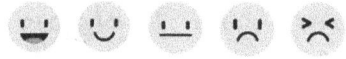

Breakfast:

_____

_____

_____

_____

Lunch:

_____

_____

_____

_____

Dinner:

_____

_____

_____

_____

Snacks:

_____

_____

_____

_____

Water: 🥛🥛🥛🥛🥛🥛🥛🥛🥛🥛🥛🥛🥛🥛🥛

How was my day?

_____

_____

_____

What could I improve tomorrow?

_____

_____

_____

Reflection - Week 9

How was my week?

_____

_____

_____

_____

_____

What lesson did I learn?

_____

_____

_____

_____

_____

What change would make next
week (even) better?

_____

_____

_____

_____

_____

FOOD IDEAS - Week 10

Breakfast:

Lunch:

Dinner:

Snacks:

SHOPPING LIST - Week 10

Day (64)

How did I sleep?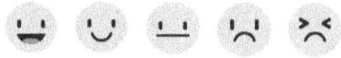

Breakfast:

_____
_____
_____
_____

Lunch:

_____
_____
_____
_____

Dinner:

_____
_____
_____
_____

Snacks:

_____
_____
_____
_____

Water: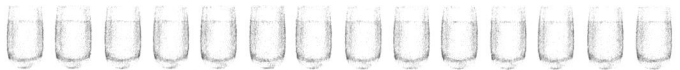

How was my day?

_____
_____
_____

What could I improve tomorrow?

_____
_____
_____

How did I sleep?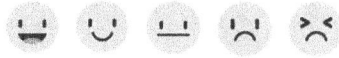

Breakfast:

Lunch:

Dinner:

Snacks:

Water: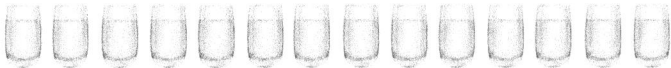

How was my day?

What could I improve tomorrow?

Day (66)

How did I sleep?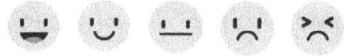

Breakfast: Lunch:

_____   _____

_____   _____

_____   _____

_____   _____

Dinner: Snacks:

_____   _____

_____   _____

_____   _____

Water:

How was my day?

_____

_____

_____

What could I improve tomorrow?

_____

_____

_____

Day (67)

How did I sleep? 😀 🙂 😐 🙁 😣

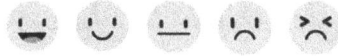

Breakfast: Lunch:

_____   _____

_____   _____

_____   _____

Dinner: Snacks:

_____   _____

_____   _____

_____   _____

Water: ⊔⊔⊔⊔⊔⊔⊔⊔⊔⊔⊔⊔⊔⊔

How was my day?

_____

_____

What could I improve tomorrow?

_____

_____

Day 68

How did I sleep?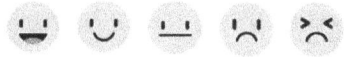

Breakfast:

_____
_____
_____
_____

Lunch:

_____
_____
_____
_____

Dinner:

_____
_____
_____

Snacks:

_____
_____
_____

Water: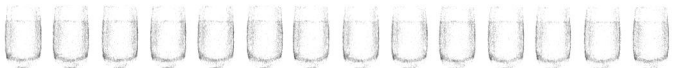

How was my day?

_____
_____
_____

What could I improve tomorrow?

_____
_____
_____

How did I sleep? 😀 🙂 😐 🙁 😣

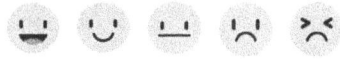

Breakfast:

Lunch:

Dinner:

Snacks:

Water:

How was my day?

What could I improve tomorrow?

Day 70

How did I sleep?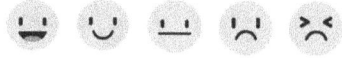

Breakfast:

_____
_____
_____
_____

Lunch:

_____
_____
_____
_____

Dinner:

_____
_____
_____
_____

Snacks:

_____
_____
_____
_____

Water: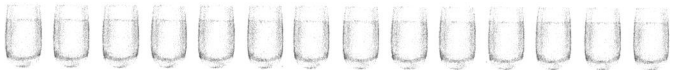

How was my day?

_____
_____
_____

What could I improve tomorrow?

_____
_____
_____

Reflection - Week 10

How was my week?

_____

_____

_____

_____

What lesson did I learn?

_____

_____

_____

_____

What change would make next
week (even) better?

_____

_____

_____

_____

FOOD IDEAS - Week 11

Breakfast:

Lunch:

Dinner:

Snacks:

SHOPPING LIST - Week 11

Day (71)

How did I sleep?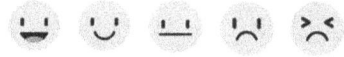

Breakfast: Lunch:

Dinner: Snacks:

Water: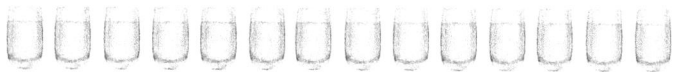

How was my day?

What could I improve tomorrow?

Day (72)

How did I sleep?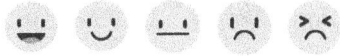

Breakfast: Lunch:

_____   _____
_____   _____
_____   _____

Dinner: Snacks:

_____   _____
_____   _____
_____   _____

Water: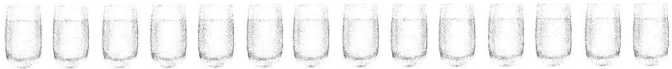

How was my day?

_____
_____

What could I improve tomorrow?

_____
_____

Day (73)

How did I sleep?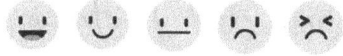

Breakfast:

_____
_____
_____
_____

Lunch:

_____
_____
_____
_____

Dinner:

_____
_____
_____
_____

Snacks:

_____
_____
_____
_____

Water: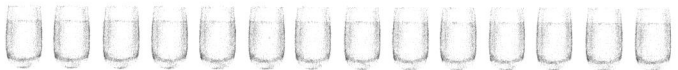

How was my day?

_____
_____
_____

What could I improve tomorrow?

_____
_____
_____

How did I sleep?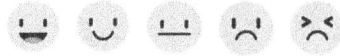

Breakfast:

_____
_____
_____
_____

Lunch:

_____
_____
_____
_____

Dinner:

_____
_____
_____
_____

Snacks:

_____
_____
_____
_____

Water: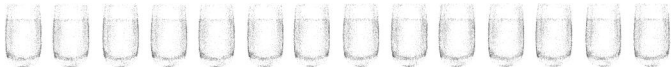

How was my day?

_____
_____
_____

What could I improve tomorrow?

_____
_____

Day (75)

How did I sleep?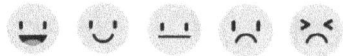

Breakfast:

Lunch:

Dinner:

Snacks:

Water: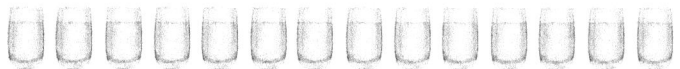

How was my day?

What could I improve tomorrow?

Day (76)

How did I sleep?   😃 🙂 😐 🙁 😖

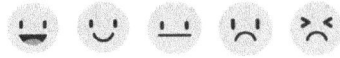

Breakfast:

_____
_____
_____
_____

Lunch:

_____
_____
_____
_____

Dinner:

_____
_____
_____
_____

Snacks:

_____
_____
_____
_____

Water: 🥛🥛🥛🥛🥛🥛🥛🥛🥛🥛🥛🥛🥛

How was my day?

_____
_____
_____

What could I improve tomorrow?

_____
_____
_____

Day (77)

How did I sleep?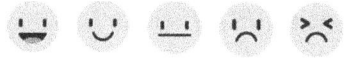

Breakfast:

_____
_____
_____
_____

Lunch:

_____
_____
_____
_____

Dinner:

_____
_____
_____

Snacks:

_____
_____
_____

Water: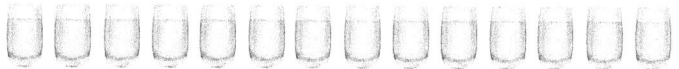

How was my day?

_____
_____
_____

What could I improve tomorrow?

_____
_____
_____

Reflection - Week 11

How was my week?

What lesson did I learn?

What change would make next week (even) better?

FOOD IDEAS - Week 12

Breakfast:

Lunch:

Dinner:

Snacks:

SHOPPING LIST - Week 12

Day (78)

How did I sleep?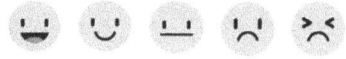

Breakfast:

Lunch:

Dinner:

Snacks:

Water: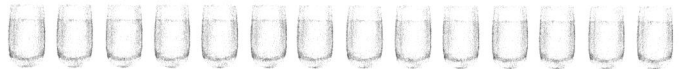

How was my day?

What could I improve tomorrow?

How did I sleep?

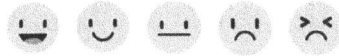

Breakfast:

_____
_____
_____
_____

Lunch:

_____
_____
_____
_____

Dinner:

_____
_____
_____
_____

Snacks:

_____
_____
_____
_____

Water:

How was my day?

_____
_____
_____

What could I improve tomorrow?

_____
_____
_____

Day 80

How did I sleep?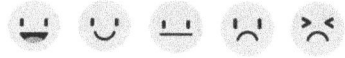

Breakfast:

_____
_____
_____
_____

Lunch:

_____
_____
_____
_____

Dinner:

_____
_____
_____

Snacks:

_____
_____
_____

Water: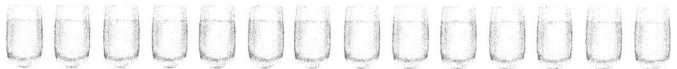

How was my day?

_____
_____
_____

What could I improve tomorrow?

_____
_____

Day (81)

How did I sleep?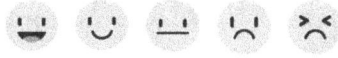

Breakfast:

Lunch:

_____
_____
_____
_____

_____
_____
_____
_____

Dinner:

Snacks:

_____
_____
_____
_____

_____
_____
_____
_____

Water: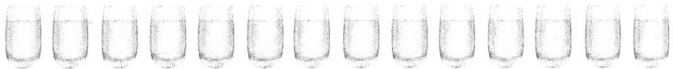

How was my day?

_____
_____
_____

What could I improve tomorrow?

_____
_____
_____

Day (82)

How did I sleep?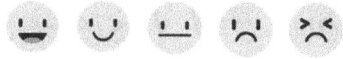

Breakfast:

_____
_____
_____
_____

Lunch:

_____
_____
_____
_____

Dinner:

_____
_____
_____
_____

Snacks:

_____
_____
_____
_____

Water: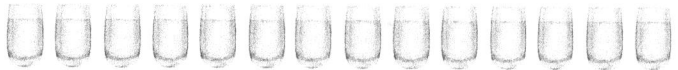

How was my day?

_____
_____
_____

What could I improve tomorrow?

_____
_____
_____

How did I sleep?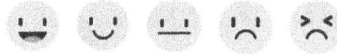

Breakfast: Lunch:

Dinner: Snacks:

Water: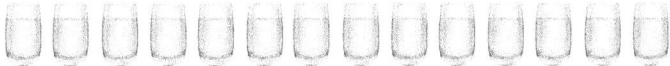

How was my day?

What could I improve tomorrow?

Day (84)

How did I sleep? 😃 🙂 😐 🙁 😣

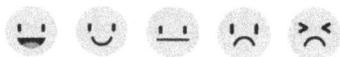

Breakfast:

Lunch:

Dinner:

Snacks:

Water: ⎍⎍⎍⎍⎍⎍⎍⎍⎍⎍⎍⎍⎍⎍

How was my day?

What could I improve tomorrow?

Reflection - Week 12

How was my week?

What lesson did I learn?

What change would make next
week (even) better?

Stats After 12 Weeks:

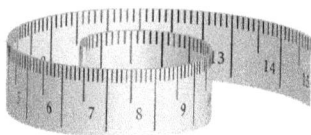

Weight: _____

Chest: _____

Arm: _____

Waist: _____

Hips: _____

Thigh: _____

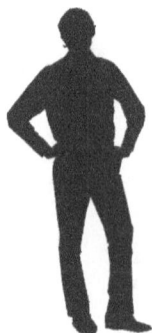 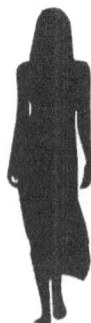

Want to keep going?

You are (almost) at the end of this meal planner.

Well done!

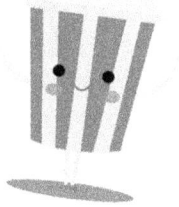

But...you're about to run out of space. And you may want to continue with your meal tracking habit.

Don't worry!

On the next pages, you will find a **BONUS** week. This gives you time to get your hands on a new planner.

Let's continue.

FOOD IDEAS - Week 13

Breakfast:

Lunch:

Dinner:

Snacks:

SHOPPING LIST - Week 13

Day (85)

How did I sleep? 😃 🙂 😐 🙁 😣

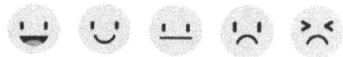

Breakfast:

_____

_____

_____

_____

Lunch:

_____

_____

_____

_____

Dinner:

_____

_____

_____

_____

Snacks:

_____

_____

_____

_____

Water: ⎕⎕⎕⎕⎕⎕⎕⎕⎕⎕⎕⎕⎕⎕⎕

How was my day?

_____

_____

_____

What could I improve tomorrow?

_____

_____

_____

How did I sleep?　😀 🙂 😐 🙁 😣

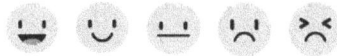

Breakfast:

_____
_____
_____
_____

Lunch:

_____
_____
_____
_____

Dinner:

_____
_____
_____

Snacks:

_____
_____
_____

Water: 🥛🥛🥛🥛🥛🥛🥛🥛🥛🥛🥛🥛🥛🥛

How was my day?

_____
_____
_____

What could I improve tomorrow?

_____
_____
_____

Day (87)

How did I sleep?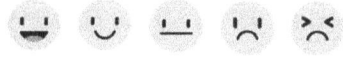

Breakfast:
_____
_____
_____
_____

Lunch:
_____
_____
_____
_____

Dinner:
_____
_____
_____

Snacks:
_____
_____
_____

Water: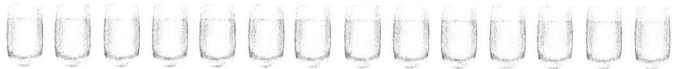

How was my day?
_____
_____
_____

What could I improve tomorrow?
_____
_____

Day (88)

How did I sleep?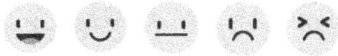

Breakfast:

_____

Lunch:

_____

Dinner:

_____

Snacks:

_____

Water: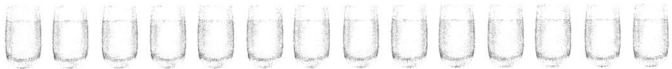

How was my day?

_____

What could I improve tomorrow?

_____

Day (89)

How did I sleep?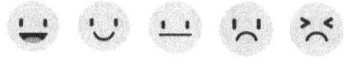

Breakfast:

Lunch:

Dinner:

Snacks:

Water: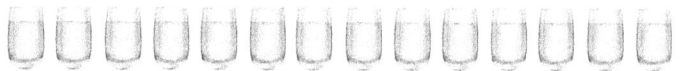

How was my day?

What could I improve tomorrow?

Day (90)

How did I sleep?

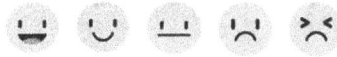

Breakfast:

_____
_____
_____
_____

Lunch:

_____
_____
_____
_____

Dinner:

_____
_____
_____
_____

Snacks:

_____
_____
_____
_____

Water:

How was my day?

_____
_____
_____

What could I improve tomorrow?

_____
_____
_____

Day 91

How did I sleep? 😀 🙂 😐 🙁 😣

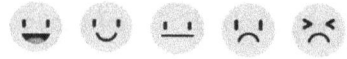

Breakfast:

_____
_____
_____
_____

Lunch:

_____
_____
_____
_____

Dinner:

_____
_____
_____

Snacks:

_____
_____
_____

Water: ⎕⎕⎕⎕⎕⎕⎕⎕⎕⎕⎕⎕⎕⎕

How was my day?

_____
_____
_____

What could I improve tomorrow?

_____
_____
_____

Reflection - Week 13

How was my week?

_____

_____

_____

_____

_____

What lesson did I learn?

_____

_____

_____

_____

What change would make next
week (even) better?

_____

_____

_____

_____

BOOM: You Did It!

Congratulations: You tracked your meals for a whopping **3 months!**

You are **AWESOME!**

Did you achieve the goal you set for yourself? You must have had a **strong WHY** to stay on course.

Is this where it ends?

No. This is only the beginning. The beginning of a new **YOU**. It's much harder to get started than to keep going.

You have now developed this amazing habit of eating healthy and keeping your weight in check. You can do anything you set your mind to.

So, what's next for you?

Don't wait for the

Perfect Moment

Take the moment

AND

Make It

Perfect

Did you like this Meal Planner?

If you enjoyed this meal planner, I would like to ask you for a favor.

Could you please leave a review online?

Reviews are the lifeblood of independent authors. I know, you're short on time. But I would really appreciate even just a few sentences!

The more reviews this meal planner gets, the more people will be able to find it and improve their health by tracking what they eat.

Thank you again for using this meal planner. Good luck with staying fit and healthy!

I'm rooting for you...